Cambridge Elements

Elements in Emergency Neurosurgery
edited by
Nihal Gurusinghe
Lancashire Teaching Hospital NHS Trust
Peter Hutchinson
University of Cambridge, Society of British Neurological Surgeons
and Royal College of Surgeons of England
Ioannis Fouyas
Royal College of Surgeons of Edinburgh
Naomi Slator
North Bristol NHS Trust
Ian Kamaly-Asl
Royal Manchester Children's Hospital
Peter Whitfield
University Hospitals Plymouth NHS Trust

MANAGEMENT OF MODERATE OR SEVERE TRAUMATIC BRAIN INJURY

Saeed Kayhanian
University of Cambridge

Erta Beqiri
University of Cambridge

Ari Ercole
University of Cambridge

Adel Helmy
University of Cambridge

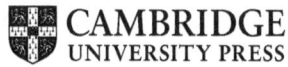

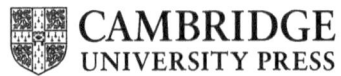

Shaftesbury Road, Cambridge CB2 8EA, United Kingdom

One Liberty Plaza, 20th Floor, New York, NY 10006, USA

477 Williamstown Road, Port Melbourne, VIC 3207, Australia

314–321, 3rd Floor, Plot 3, Splendor Forum, Jasola District Centre, New Delhi – 110025, India

103 Penang Road, #05–06/07, Visioncrest Commercial, Singapore 238467

Cambridge University Press is part of Cambridge University Press & Assessment, a department of the University of Cambridge.

We share the University's mission to contribute to society through the pursuit of education, learning and research at the highest international levels of excellence.

www.cambridge.org
Information on this title: www.cambridge.org/9781009437707
DOI: 10.1017/9781009437677

© Saeed Kayhanian, Erta Beqiri, Ari Ercole and Adel Helmy 2025

This publication is in copyright. Subject to statutory exception and to the provisions of relevant collective licensing agreements, no reproduction of any part may take place without the written permission of Cambridge University Press & Assessment.

When citing this work, please include a reference to the DOI 10.1017/9781009437677

First published 2025

A catalogue record for this publication is available from the British Library

ISBN 978-1-009-43770-7 Paperback
ISSN 2755-0656 (online)
ISSN 2755-0648 (print)

Cambridge University Press & Assessment has no responsibility for the persistence or accuracy of URLs for external or third-party internet websites referred to in this publication and does not guarantee that any content on such websites is, or will remain, accurate or appropriate.

For EU product safety concerns, contact us at Calle de José Abascal, 56, 1°, 28003 Madrid, Spain, or email eugpsr@cambridge.org

Every effort has been made in preparing this Element to provide accurate and up-to-date information which is in accord with accepted standards and practice at the time of publication. Although case histories are drawn from actual cases, every effort has been made to disguise the identities of the individuals involved. Nevertheless, the authors, editors and publishers can make no warranties that the information contained herein is totally free from error, not least because clinical standards are constantly changing through research and regulation. The authors, editors and publishers therefore disclaim all liability for direct or consequential damages resulting from the use of material contained in this Element. Readers are strongly advised to pay careful attention to information provided by the manufacturer of any drugs or equipment that they plan to use.

Management of Moderate or Severe Traumatic Brain Injury

Elements in Emergency Neurosurgery

DOI: 10.1017/9781009437677
First published online: May 2025

Saeed Kayhanian
University of Cambridge

Erta Beqiri
University of Cambridge

Ari Ercole
University of Cambridge

Adel Helmy
University of Cambridge

Author for correspondence: Saeed Kayhanian, sk776@cam.ac.uk

Abstract: The management of patients with moderate and severe traumatic brain injury (TBI) is centred on the intensive care management to limit the extent of secondary injury to the brain, following the primary trauma. This management aims to optimise the homeostatic environment of the brain after injury and can be guided by multimodality monitoring, including intracranial pressure (ICP) monitoring. This management often follows a tiered approach to introducing more aggressive interventions to correct physiology, based on evidence for ongoing secondary injury, such as raised ICP. The balance between risk and benefit for these interventions for individual patients is difficult, particularly in the absence of high-quality randomised trials for many interventions in this area. In this Element, the authors outline both the approach to intensive care management of moderate and severe TBI, as well as the evidence base available for the interventions discussed.

Keywords: traumatic brain injury, intracranial pressure, intensive care, decompressive craniectomy, cerebral perfusion pressure

© Saeed Kayhanian, Erta Beqiri, Ari Ercole and Adel Helmy 2025

ISBNs: 9781009437707 (PB), 9781009437677 (OC)
ISSNs: 2755-0656 (online), 2755-0648 (print)

Contents

Intensive Care Management – General Measures   1

ICP   8

Tiered ICP Management Strategy   11

Multimodality Monitoring   13

Conclusion   17

References   18

Intensive Care Management – General Measures

Goal

The severity of traumatic brain injury (TBI) is usually classified based on a patient's Glasgow Coma Scale (GCS) score after initial resuscitation, with a GCS score of 9–13 graded as moderate and a score <9 graded as severe TBI.

Intensive care management of moderate and severe TBI aims to optimise physiology and avoid secondary insults, which may occur at any point after the admission. Current guidelines and protocols are focused on controlling intracranial pressure (ICP) and maintaining cerebral perfusion pressure (CPP) [1,2]. Specific ICP/CPP management is discussed in the section 'Tiered ICP Management Strategy' and single strategies are presented in Table 1. Here, we give an overview of general intensive care measures.

Ventilatory Strategies

Mechanical ventilation is crucial in maintaining adequate arterial partial pressure of oxygen and carbon dioxide ($PaCO_2$). Hypoxia causes hypoxic injury and hypoxic cerebral vasodilation, ultimately increasing ICP. On the other hand, (normobaric) hyperoxia can increase cerebral excitotoxicity in severe TBI and may lead to reactive oxygen species formation [3].

Early TBI is characterised by a state of ischaemia and hyperventilation/hypocapnia may exacerbate this. At the same time, hypercapnia should be avoided given its cerebral vasodilatory effect, which increases ICP particularly later on after injury as intracranial compliance decreases as cerebral oedema progresses as a result of the inflammatory response to injury. Volume-controlled ventilation allows appropriately tight control of $PaCO_2$, which should target levels at the low end of normal (4.5–5.0 kPa)

Lung protective ventilation strategies should be employed as far as is possible. Concerns are sometimes cited regarding a potentially deleterious effect of PEEP on ICP. However, this is largely theoretical (since poor lung compliance in ARDS limits the transmission of airway pressure to the circulation) and entirely outweighed by the need to maintain oxygenation. Early tracheostomy (<8 days) is thought to associate with better neurological outcome and reduced length of stay [4].

Sedation and Analgesia

Adequate sedation (with propofol or midazolam) is needed for endotracheal tube tolerance, compliance with mechanical ventilation, and also reduces cerebral metabolic rate. A combination of hypnotic and opioid (such as

Table 1 ICP management strategies

Strategy	Mechanism of action/advantages/recommendations	How to monitor	Targets	Risks and disadvantages
Hyperventilation	- Hypocapnia causes vasoconstriction, which can result in desired reduction of ICP in cases of raised ICP and low brain compliance. - The effect on ICP would be transient, given the renormalisation of extravascular pH that follows prolonged hypocapnia.	pCO2, rsO2	4–4.5 KPa	When ICP levels are within normal range or when hypocapnia is prolonged, the effects of hypocapnia are mainly reflected in undesired cerebral ischemia.
Sedation	- Reduces CMRO2. When used in combination with analgesia, reduces pain and agitation. - Propofol has a rapid onset and a short duration of action, and at <4 mg/kg/h preserves CBF/CMRO2 coupling, cerebrovascular reactivity and brain oxygenation. - Midazolam causes less haemodynamic instability.	Sedation-analgesia scoring tools		- Propofol tends to cause hypotension and the use of high doses for prolonged period may lead to propofol infusion syndrome. - Midazolam is less effective in controlling refractory intracranial hypertension and has disadvantages of tolerance and tachyphylaxis, and accumulation in renal dysfunction.

Analgesia	Sedation-analgesia scoring tools.	- Suppression of cough and gag reflexes, pain control - Long-acting opioids such as fentanyl or morphine allow to achieve stable and prolonged sedation which is beneficial in management of intracranial hypertension. - Remifentanil has a rapid onset and a short duration of action, which allows for neurological assessment, and the clearance is independent of renal or hepatic function.	Remifentanil is less effective in controlling raised ICP.
Targeted temperature management	Core temperature	- Mild (34.0–35.9°C) - Moderate (32.0–33.9°C)	- Hypothermia leads to a decrease in the metabolic rate and thus decreases cerebral oedema and neuronal apoptosis. - Targeted temperature management to avoid fever has been shown superior to induced hypothermia.	- Increase in ABP, decrease in HR and CO. - Increase in PR and QT interval and QRS complex (arrhythmia develop at <30 °C) - Decrease in K, Mg, P, Ca. Increase in K during rewarming - Leucopenia, thrombocytopenia, hyperglycaemia, increase in lactate, transaminases and amylase - Infections

Table 1 (cont.)

Strategy	Mechanism of action/advantages/recommendations	How to monitor	Targets	Risks and disadvantages
Antiepileptic drug therapy	- Seizures increase brain energy demand. - 7 days ADT as prophylaxis of early post traumatic seizures is recommended in patients with risk factors such as GCS < 10, penetrating head wound, cortical contusion, depressed skull fractures or large hematomas.	Continuous EEG monitoring may detect non-convulsive seizures		- AED therapy to prevent late post traumatic seizures is not recommended
Osmotic therapy	- Intravenous infusion of hypertonic saline or mannitol is indicated for acute rises of ICP and controls brain oedema. - Expands the plasma volume, decreases blood viscosity; after plasma osmolarity increases, the gradient across the blood-brain barrier draws water from the brain into the vascular compartment.	Na+, diuresis		- Mannitol leads to diuresis and subsequent hypovolaemia and hypotension; repeated administrations of Mannitol increase serum osmolarity

	- Hypertonic saline is not associated with subsequent diuresis and hypovolaemia and is preferred over mannitol.		
EVD	- The drainage of cerebrospinal fluid reduces cerebral volume and decreases ICP	- EVD drainage height regulated ICP and CSF flow	- Aim to keep ICP below 20 cmH$_2$O	- Small procedural morbidity from inserting EVD - Risk of infection, particularly if longer than 5 days in situ
Decompressive craniectomy	- Part of the skull is removed to accommodate brain swelling (brain compliance increases)	- Bulging/tense flap	- Aim to keep ICP below 20 cmH$_2$O	- Procedural risks - Need for further procedure (cranioplasty) - CSF flow problems - Syndrome of the Trephined

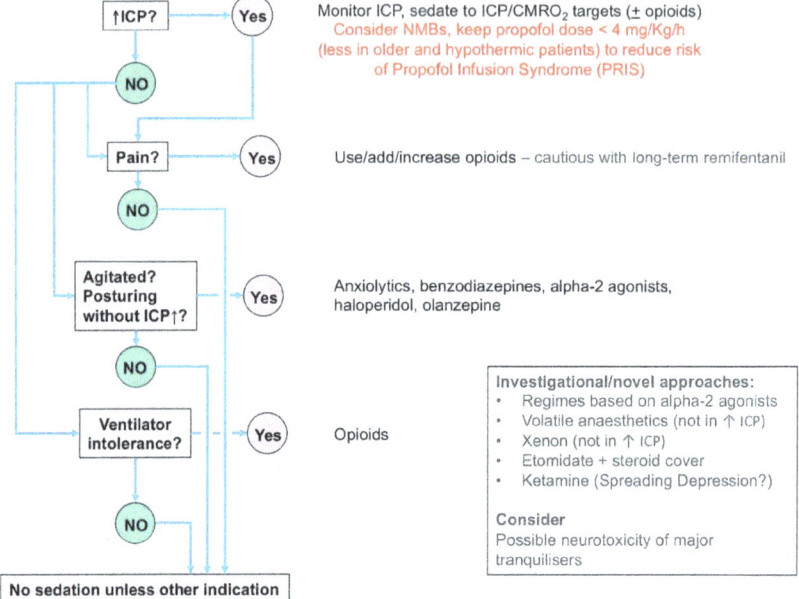

Figure 1 Practical approach to sedation-analgesia

fentanyl, morphine or remifentanil) infusions is typically used as this controls cough and gag reflexes, controls pain aiding ICP control (see Table 1). Infusions of neuromuscular blockers may be needed as an adjunct.

Agitation and delirium during the period of emergence from sedation can be treated with anxiolytics such as benzodiazepines, neuroleptics and α2-agonists such as clonidine and dexmedetomidine as well as attention to providing adequate analgesia for extracranial injuries. Evidence is limited but a pragmatic approach to the management of sedation-analgesia is shown in Figure 1.

Haemodynamic Support

Haemodynamic stability should be achieved as soon as possible after TBI in order to ensure adequate cerebral oxygen delivery. The cardiovascular system management can be challenging in TBI patients variously because of haemorrhage from extracranial injuries, concomitant myocardial injury, or fluid balance problems such as diabetes insipidus. Hypotension causes detrimental cerebral hypoperfusion and ischemia, while hypertension runs the risk of driving cerebral oedema and ultimately increasing ICP, particularly if autoregulation is impaired.

Isotonic crystalloids can be used for fluid resuscitation aiming for euvolemia, carefully avoiding hyponatremia. Disruptions of the osmotic gradient across the brain-blood barrier can lead to brain oedema and an increase in ICP. Vasopressors such as noradrenaline or phenylephrine can support CPP as required. Hypotonic fluids should be avoided.

Haemoglobin concentration is a balance between oxygen delivery and blood viscosity compromising microcirculatory flow. Transfusion thresholds after TBI are controversial and should be individualised according to the prevailing physiology, but transfusion targets between 8 and 10 g/dL are commonly employed in practice.

Management of haemostatic defects after TBI may be guided by viscoelastic tests and platelet function tests. Major haemorrhage from extracranial injuries is common and warrants resuscitation with blood/FFP and damage control surgery as appropriate. Fibrinogen should be maintained >1.5 g/L. Platelet count should be $>100 \times 10^9$/L in the acute phase for both neurosurgical procedures and avoidance of haemorrhage progression.

High rates of venous thromboembolism (VTE) are associated with TBI, and trauma in general. Low molecular weight heparin or low-dose unfractionated heparin may be used in combination with mechanical prophylaxis. In patients with haemorrhagic lesions, VTE chemoprophylaxis can be initiated at 24–72 hours if there is no evidence of haematoma progression at repeated neuroimaging. In patients who do show evidence of lesion progression, VTE prophylaxis can be delayed, and this question is currently the focus of a large randomised trial (TOP-TBI).

Metabolic Support

A state of hypermetabolism and hypercatabolism is common after trauma and therefore enteral nutrition should start within 48 hours, aiming for full caloric supplementation by 7 days. Stress ulcer prophylaxis (e.g. with a PPI) is standard practice at least until full enteral feeding is achieved.

Tight systemic glucose control is associated with reduced cerebral extracellular glucose availability and increased prevalence of brain energy crisis. Current management focuses on avoiding hyperglycaemia without risking hypoglycaemia, with a blood glucose target of 4–10 mmol/L. Glucose targets can be optimised using cerebral microdialysis (see 'Multimodality Monitoring' section) in order to avoid neuroglycopenia and metabolic distress. Alternative substrates for brain energy production are being investigated.

Dysnatraemia is common after TBI. Hyponatraemia is of particular concern as it may worsen cerebral oedema making ICP control difficult. Many textbooks refer to SIADH and 'cerebral salt wasting' as endocrine causes of hyponatraemia after acute brain syndromes such as TBI although the pathobiology is not clear cut. It is more useful to understand that endocrine dysfunction after TBI may lead either inappropriate water retention (which requires fluid restriction) or excessive urinary sodium loss (characterised by high urinary sodium and which requires sodium supplementation and/or the use of mineralocorticoids to reduce excretion), both of which cause hyponatraemia. In reality, however, fluid restriction is usually inappropriate in the acute situation as it risks hypovolaemia and infusions of hypertonic saline are the only intervention which may address life-threatening hyponatraemia in an acceptable timescale.

Posterior pituitary failure is also seen after TBI which may lead to diabetes insipidus (DI). The resulting hypernatraemia is often of lesser concern unless very severe; indeed, it is potentially very dangerous to try to correct this in the acute setting so efforts should focus on preventing worsening rather than normalising it. However, the diuresis seen in severe DI may occasionally be sufficiently torrential as to lead to dangerous hypovolaemia. Whilst DI is typically transient, treatment with desmopressin (or occasionally argipressin infusions) may be necessary. Anterior pituitary dysfunction is also recognised as common after TBI but is usually not possible to diagnose in intensive care settings.

ICP

Definition

Intracranial pressure is the pressure inside the intracranial compartment, which lays within the rigid skull and the thecal sac. For simplicity, here we will refer only to the rigid skull enclosure.

Under normal conditions and at rest, ICP remains < 15 mmHg, it fluctuates with cardiac and respiratory cycles, and has a typical P1 > P2 > P3 waveform shape (Figure 2: Box – ICP).

After TBI, CSF is displaced by oedematous brain tissue and mass lesions such as haematomas. When compensatory mechanisms are depleted, ICP rises

---

ICP Waveform

The figure in panel A shows three examples of ICP waveforms in three different pathophysiological conditions. The red dots identify the characteristic peaks P1 (percussion wave), P2 (tidal wave) and P3 (dicrotic wave), counted as they appear in chronological order. The top chart shows a normal waveform with P1 > P2 > P3 for each pulse. ICP fluctuates at low levels. The second chart shows fluctuations of ICP at higher levels. The waveform is pathological with P2 > P1, suggesting low cerebral

(cont.)

compliance. In the bottom chart, the waveform is distorted, the shape of the pulse is triangular and ICP levels are pathologically high (brain death).

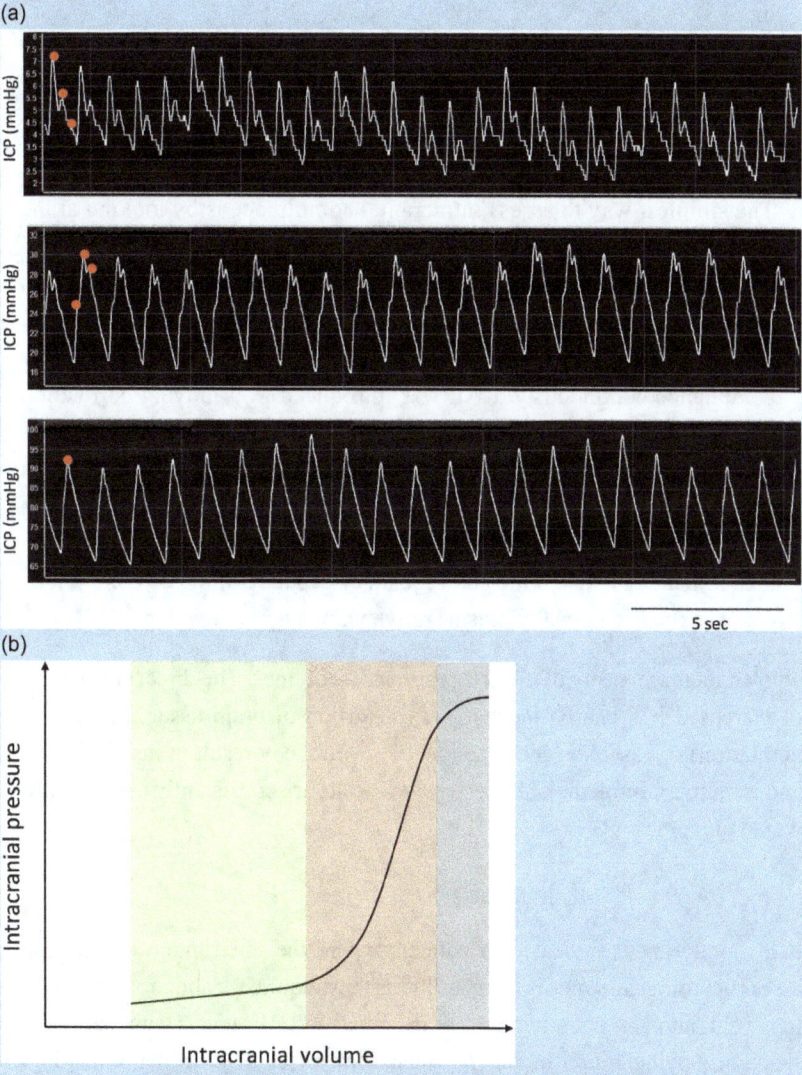

Figure 2 ICP (waveform, cerebral compliance)

Signal processing-based waveform analysis of ICP enables derivation of secondary indices, which carry information about intracranial compliance and cerebrovascular reactivity.

Intracranial Compliance and P–V Curve

Intracranial Compliance refers to the change in cerebral volume per unit change in ICP. Panel B shows a depictive pressure–volume curve for the

(cont.)

brain. A high compliance (green area) denotes the ability of the intracranial compartment to accommodate an increase in volume without a large increase in ICP.

A low intracranial compliance (red area) indicates that any further incremental volume changing insult may result in rapid escalation of ICP. The grey area corresponds to depleted cerebrovascular reactivity.

Monitoring Cerebral Compliance

The simplest way to assess intracranial compliance is by looking at the shape of the pulse waveform of ICP. Dominant P2 (second chart in panel A) or triangular shape of the pulse (bottom chart in panel A) reflects a reduced compliance.

The compensatory reserve index (RAP) can be used to monitor cerebral compliance continuously. RAP was introduced as a moving correlation coefficient between 6 or 10 seconds average pulse amplitude of ICP and mean value of ICP over 4 minutes of time. A RAP value near 1 indicates poor or exhausted compensatory reserve (red area in panel B). RAP close to 0 denotes preserved compensatory reserve at low values of ICP (green area in panel B). When the autoregulatory capacity of the cerebral arterioles is exhausted, RAP yields negative values (grey area in panel B)

with an increase in any of the compartments' volumes. The direct consequences of increased ICP can be mechanical (distortion of brain tissue, midline shift, herniation) or vascular (decrease in CPP, which may result in insufficient CBF and ischemia). Intracranial hypertensive events are consistently associated with worse outcomes.

Indication for Monitoring

ICP monitoring is indicated in patients where the interruption of sedation to assess neurological status is not possible as they require sedation for other reasons (e.g. ventilation for chest injuries), or in comatose TBI patients with clear signs of space-occupying lesion or other evidence of raised ICP on neuroimaging. In patients with normal or borderline neuroimaging but with significant extracranial injuries, and in patients where the clinical examination is not completely reliable (severe maxillofacial trauma, spinal cord injury), the options are either to place an ICP monitor or to perform further serial imaging. Individual cases should be evaluated for risks and benefits of ICP sensor insertion.

ICP monitoring provides an indication of development of pathology and can guide intensive care management (see 'Tiered ICP management' paragraph).

Tiered ICP Management Strategy

The management of ICP after moderate and severe TBI is guided in many centres around the world by a tiered intervention protocol. This makes rational use of the available strategies for managing ICP, typically with the interventions that are least invasive and/or with the best evidence base appearing earlier in the algorithm. One example of such a protocol, in use at Cambridge University Hospitals, is summarised in Figure 3. Importantly, consideration should be given at each stage that any change or difficulty in controlling ICP may be caused by a new or evolving pathology that is amenable to surgical intervention and there should thus be a low threshold for repeat CT imaging to search for this. Table 1 summarises single strategies involved in the management of ICP.

Medical Interventions

Osmotic Therapy

Hyperosmotic agents can be administered as an effective short-term measure to reduce ICP. Hypertonic saline may be preferred to mannitol as it is not associated with the diuresis and potential subsequent hypovolaemia and hypotension that can result after mannitol administration. The use of hypertonic saline over mannitol is supported by evidence from small comparative trials but definitive, high-quality evidence is lacking [5]. The Sugar or Salt (SoS) randomised trial is currently recruiting to address this question.

Temperature Management

Targeted temperature management used to avoid fever may confer benefits in controlling ICP but the results of the trial Eurotherm3235 suggest that harm from early therapeutic hypothermia for patients with ICP > 20 outweighs benefit [6]. There may be scope for the use of therapeutic hypothermia as a rescue therapy as this is an effective strategy for controlling ICP but the evidence of beneficial outcomes remains very limited. Changes in drug metabolism with hypothermia are a concern: propofol dosing should be limited (by introduction of other sedatives) because of the theoretically increased risk of propofol infusion syndrome.

Seizure Management

Patients with TBI are at high risk of seizures, with up to one-third demonstrating non-convulsive seizure activity on continuous EEG monitoring. Seven days of anti-epileptic drug (AED) therapy are recommended in TBI patients at particularly high risk of seizures (GCS < 10, penetrating head wound, cortical contusion, depressed skull fractures or large hematomas). The use of levetiracetam

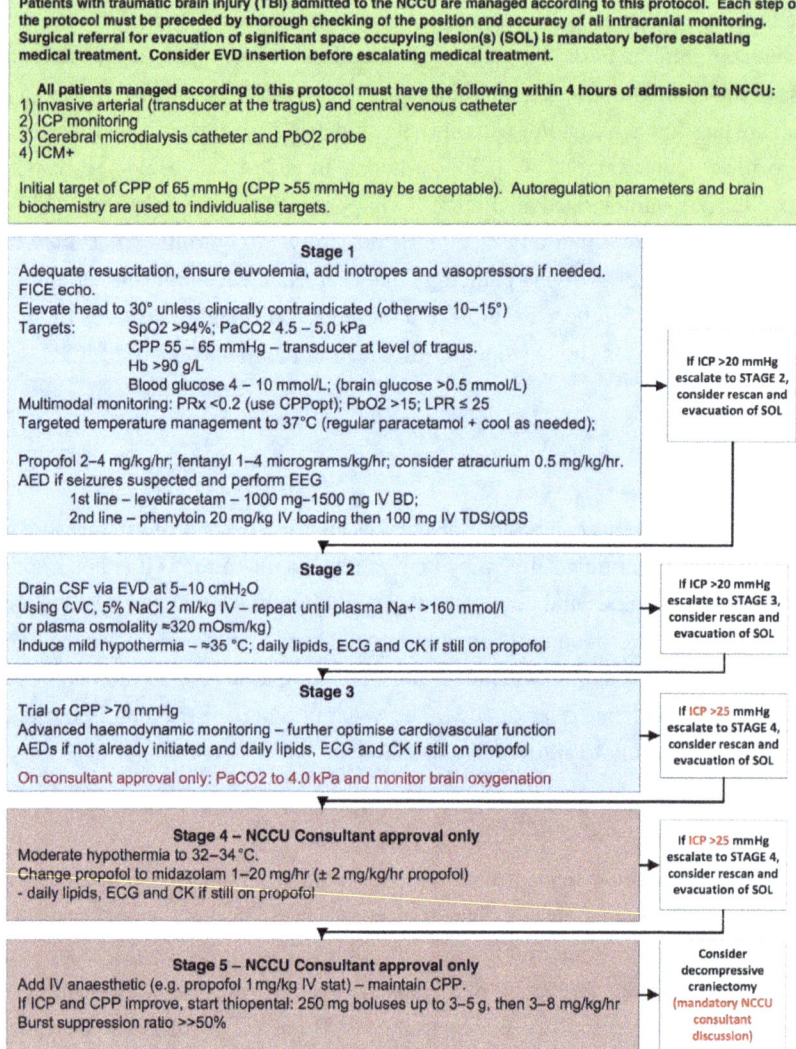

Figure 3 ICP/CPP management algorithm

may be preferred over phenytoin due to its favourable safety profile. The use and choice of prophylactic AEDs after TBI are currently the subject of a large, multi-centre randomised trial (MAST).

Barbiturate Coma

The use of barbiturates to achieve deep sedation (burst suppression) may be used as a final line rescue intervention to manage refractory ICP. Barbiturates

Management of Moderate or Severe Traumatic Brain Injury

suppress cerebral metabolism and are effective in lowering ICP, but carry significant risks including respiratory complications, hepatic and renal impairment, as well as haemodynamic instability and hypotension which may increase mortality in TBI patients.

Surgical Interventions

Surgical management of moderate and severe TBI aims to mitigate injury through evacuation of haematomas and/or the management of refractory ICP (see chapter 35). For the management of ICP, the results from two randomised control trials suggest that early decompressive craniectomy for moderate intracranial hypertension does not improve outcomes after TBI (DECRA trial) whereas 'late' intervention for persistent ICP > 25 mmHg results in increased survival at 12 months, though with increased numbers of survivors with severe disability, as compared to medical management (RESCUEicp trial) [7,8].

Multimodality Monitoring

Clinical pathophysiology and trajectory of TBI are highly heterogeneous. A multimodality approach, both invasive and non-invasive, can describe and track pathophysiology in real-time, allowing for precision medicine strategies [9,10]. Table 2 presents normal ranges and thresholds used for the treatment of multimodality monitoring derived variables.

Cerebral Autoregulation

Continuous monitoring of cerebral autoregulation (CA) can provide information for individualising CPP targets (Figure 4: Box – Cerebral Autoregulation). The most validated autoregulation index is the PRx. A positive index indicates increases (or decreases) in arterial blood pressure (ABP) causing increase (or

Table 2 Multimodality monitoring derived thresholds

	Normal range	Threshold for injury/treatment	
		Less stringent	More stringent
ICP	<15 mmHg	20–25 mmHg	20 mmHg
PRx	<0.0	>0.3	>0.0
$P_{bt}O2$	~30 mmHg	15–20 mmHg	<15 mmHg
LPR	<25	>25	>40
Brain tissue glucose	1–2 mmol/L	<0.8 mmol/L	<0.2 mmol/L

ICP: Intracranial pressure; PRx: pressure reactivity index; $P_{bt}O2$: tissue oxygen tension; LPR: lactate:pyruvate ratio.

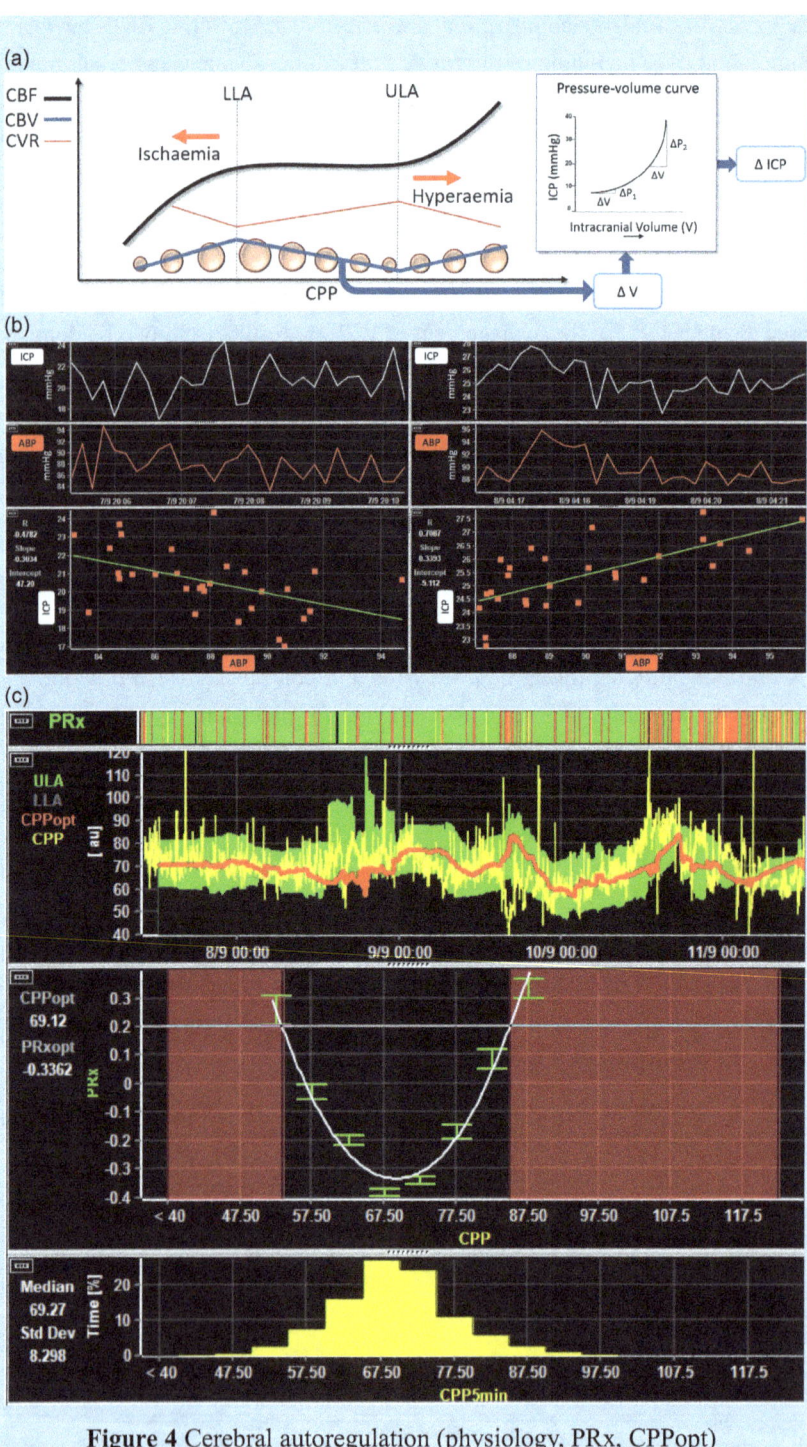

Figure 4 Cerebral autoregulation (physiology, PRx, CPPopt)

Physiology

Panel A shows the cerebral autoregulatory curve (left part of the figure). There is a range of CPP values where, thanks to active vasoconstriction and vasodilation of cerebral arteriola (red circles in the figure), autoregulation minimises fluctuations in cerebral blood flow (CBF) driven by variations in ICP and/or ABP. Outside of the autoregulatory range, the relationship between pressure and flow becomes more passive. This leads to increased risk of both ischaemia, at low CPP, or hyperaemia, at high CPP.

Pressure Reactivity Index

Changes in vessels diameters are reflected into fluctuations in cerebral blood volume (panel A) which are transmitted into slow changes in ICP according to the pressure-volume curve of the brain (right part of the figure). Hence, the cerebrovascular reactivity can be assessed by measuring how vasogenic changes in ABP are transmitted to ICP. The pressure reactivity index (PRx) relies on this principle.

PRx can be calculated in a semi-continuous manner by a monitoring software at the bedside as a moving correlation of 30 consecutive 10-second averages of ABP and ICP. In panel B, ICP and ABP are coarse-grained with a 10-second moving average filter. The right part of the panel, shows a negative correlation between ABP and ICP over 5 minutes, suggesting preserved autoregulation. A positive index (left part of panel B) indicates increases (or decreases) in ABP causes increase (or decrease) in blood volume and therefore ICP. Autoregulation in this case is impaired as the vessels passively dilate (or constrict). PRx is often displayed at the bedside as a risk bar chart (top chart in panel C) where red indicates lost autoregulation.

CPPopt and Limits of Autoregulation

The relationship between PRx and CPP over long periods of time often shows a U-shaped relationship (panel C, third chart). The CPP value at which PRx is more negative (corresponding to CA best preserved) is considered the optimal CPP, or CPPopt. The red area in the chart highlights CPP and PRx values outside the range of autoregulation, defined with a high PRx threshold.

It is also possible to track CPPopt and the limits of autoregulation as minute-by-minute time trends (panel C, second chart).

decrease) in blood volume and therefore ICP. Autoregulation in this case is impaired as the vessels passively dilate (or constrict). Conversely, a negative PRx represents preserved vascular reactivity.

The relationship between PRx and CPP over long periods of time often shows a U-shaped relationship. The CPP value at which PRx is more negative (corresponding to CA best preserved) is considered the optimal CPP, or CPPopt. TBI patients are at higher risk of mortality when CPP is managed below CPPopt, and disability when CPP is managed above CPPopt. COGiTATE phase II trial showed that it is feasible and safe to target CPP at CPPopt in TBI patients [11]. This is a promising strategy for protecting the brain against secondary injuries from sudden variations blood flow.

Besides PRx, flow-based and non-invasive solutions for monitoring CA include NIRS-derived Cerebral oximetry index (TOx or COx) and TCD-derived Mean velocity index (Mx). They are less validated than PRx in the realm of TBI.

Brain Oxygenation

Brain oxygenation can be assessed by direct measurement of tissue oxygen tension ($P_{bt}O_2$) using invasive monitoring probes. The rationale for this measurement alongside ICP and CPP monitoring reflects the potential for cerebral hypoxia despite unimpaired CBF, as a result of impaired oxygen diffusion in the brain parenchyma after injury. $P_{bt}O_2$-guided therapies may include interventions to improve oxygen delivery (reduce ICP, improve CBF or increase Hb). Increasing FiO_2 will cause an apparent increase in $P_{bt}O_2$ but does not improve cerebral oxygen delivery to any meaningful extent and the resultant hyperoxia may be harmful. A recent meta-analysis of three RCTs of $P_{bt}O_2$-guided management suggested no significant association with improved outcomes, though noted the available evidence was of very low quality [12]. The recently published OXY-TC multi-centre, randomised superiority trial found no benefit to $P_{bt}O_2$-guided management compared with ICP monitoring alone in severe TBI [13]. Two further RCTs of $P_{bt}O_2$-guided management strategies (BONAZA and BOOST-3) are currently ongoing.

Cerebral Microdialysis

Cerebral microdialysis uses an invasive probe to sample the extracellular space of the brain parenchyma. A perfusate is passed through a coaxial intraparenchymal catheter with a semipermeable membrane, allowing for the recovery of small molecules (typically of <20 kDa) in the effluent that reflects the local brain chemistry. Common microdialysis measurements after TBI include brain tissue glucose and the lactate:pyruvate ratio (LPR), sensitive to metabolic derangements in the brain tissue. Both low cerebral glucose and a raised LPR have been associated with worse outcomes [14].

Conclusion

The current management of moderate and severe TBI is based on a rational approach to the management of acute physiology, guided by monitoring of physiological parameters that are considered to be important to the homeostasis of the brain environment. The majority of individual interventions are underpinned by relatively weak evidence from limited observational studies but there is a growing body of randomised trial evidence. Further work is needed in this area to develop the evidence base for specific interventions, as well as to develop novel biomarkers that may help to guide a more precise approach to intervention.

References

[1] Carney N, Totten AM, Ullman JS, et al. Guidelines for the Management of Severe Traumatic Brain Injury 4th ed. 2016.

[2] Hawryluk GWJ, Aguilera S, Buki A, et al. A Management Algorithm for Patients with Intracranial Pressure Monitoring: The Seattle International Severe Traumatic Brain Injury Consensus Conference (SIBICC). Intensive Care Med. 2019;45:1783–94. https://doi.org/10.1007/S00134-019-05805-9.

[3] Singer M, Young PJ, Laffey JG, et al. Dangers of Hyperoxia. Crit. Care 2021;25:1–15. https://doi.org/10.1186/S13054-021-03815-Y.

[4] De Franca SA, Tavares WM, Salinet ASM, Paiva WS, Teixeira MJ. Early Tracheostomy in Severe Traumatic Brain Injury Patients: A Meta-Analysis and Comparison with Late Tracheostomy. Crit. Care Med. 2020;48:E325–31. https://doi.org/10.1097/CCM.0000000000004239.

[5] Li M, Chen T, Chen S Da, Cai J, Hu YH. Comparison of Equimolar Doses of Mannitol and Hypertonic Saline for the Treatment of Elevated Intracranial Pressure after Traumatic Brain Injury: A Systematic Review and Meta-Analysis. Medicine 2015;94:e668. https://doi.org/10.1097/MD.0000000000000668.

[6] Andrews PJD, Sinclair HL, Rodríguez A, et al. Therapeutic Hypothermia to Reduce Intracranial Pressure after Traumatic Brain Injury: the Eurotherm3235 RCT. Health Technol Assess (Rockv) 2018;22:1–133. https://doi.org/10.3310/HTA22450.

[7] Cooper DJ, Rosenfeld J V, Murray L, et al. Decompressive Craniectomy in Diffuse Traumatic Brain Injury. N. Engl. J. Med. 2011;364:1493–502. https://doi.org/10.1056/NEJMoa1102077.

[8] Hutchinson PJ, Kolias AG, Timofeev IS, et al. Trial of Decompressive Craniectomy for Traumatic Intracranial Hypertension. N. Engl. J. Med. 2016;375:1119–30. https://doi.org/10.1056/NEJMOA1605215/SUPPL_FILE/NEJMOA1605215_DISCLOSURES.PDF.

[9] Khellaf A, Khan DZ, Helmy A. Recent Advances in Traumatic Brain Injury. J. Neurol. 2019;266:2878–89. https://doi.org/10.1007/S00415-019-09541-4.

[10] Yang MT. Multimodal Neurocritical Monitoring. Biomed. J. 2020;43:226–30. https://doi.org/10.1016/J.BJ.2020.05.005.

[11] Tas J, Beqiri E, van Kaam CR, et al. An Update on the COGiTATE Phase II Study: Feasibility and Safety of Targeting an Optimal Cerebral Perfusion Pressure as a Patient-Tailored Therapy in Severe Traumatic Brain Injury.

Acta Neurochir. Suppl. 2021;131:143–7. https://doi.org/10.1007/978-3-030-59436-7_29.

[12] Hays LMC, Udy A, Adamides AA, et al. Effects of Brain Tissue Oxygen (PbtO2) Guided Management on Patient Outcomes Following Severe Traumatic Brain Injury: A Systematic Review and Meta-analysis. J. Clin. Neurosci. 2022;99:349–58. https://doi.org/10.1016/J.JOCN.2022.03.017.

[13] Payen JF, Launey Y, Chabanne R, et al. Intracranial Pressure Monitoring with and without Brain Tissue Oxygen Pressure Monitoring for Severe Traumatic Brain Injury in France (OXY-TC): An Open-Label, Randomised Controlled Superiority Trial. Lancet Neurol. 2023;22:1005–14. https://doi.org/10.1016/S1474-4422(23)00290-9.

[14] Timofeev I, Carpenter KLH, Nortje J, et al. Cerebral Extracellular Chemistry and Outcome Following Traumatic Brain Injury: A Microdialysis Study of 223 Patients. Brain 2011;134:484–94. https://doi.org/10.1093/BRAIN/AWQ353.

Cambridge Elements

Emergency Neurosurgery

Nihal Gurusinghe
Lancashire Teaching Hospital NHS Trust

Professor Nihal Gurusinghe is a Consultant Neurosurgeon at the Lancashire Teaching Hospitals NHS Trust. He is on the Executive Council of the Society of British Neurological Surgeons as the Lead for NICE (National Institute for Health and Care Excellence) guidelines relating to neurosurgical practice. He is also an examiner for the UK and International FRCS examinations in Neurosurgery.

Peter Hutchinson
University of Cambridge, Society of British Neurological Surgeons and Royal College of Surgeons of England

Peter Hutchinson BSc MBBS FFSEM FRCS(SN) PhD FMedSci is Professor of Neurosurgery and Head of the Division of Academic Neurosurgery at the University of Cambridge, and Honorary Consultant Neurosurgeon at Addenbrooke's Hospital. He is Director of Clinical Research at the Royal College of Surgeons of England and Meetings Secretary of the Society of British Neurological Surgeons.

Ioannis Fouyas
Royal College of Surgeons of Edinburgh

Ioannis Fouyas is a Consultant Neurosurgeon in Edinburgh. His clinical interests focus on the treatment of complex cerebrovascular and skull base pathologies. His academic endeavours concentrate in the field of cerebrovascular pathophysiology. His passion is technical surgical training, fulfilled in collaboration with the Royal College of Surgeons of Edinburgh. Finally, he pursues Undergraduate Neuroscience teaching, with a particular focus on functional Neuroanatomy.

Naomi Slator
North Bristol NHS Trust

Naomi Slator FRCS (SN) is a Consultant Spinal Neurosurgeon based at North Bristol NHS Trust. She has a specialist interest in Complex Spine alongside Cranial and Spinal Trauma. She completed her neurosurgical training in Birmingham and a six-month Fellowship in CSF and Trauma (2019). She then went on to complete her Spinal Fellowship in Leeds (2020) before moving to the southwest to take up her consultant post.

Ian Kamaly-Asl
Royal Manchester Children's Hospital

Ian Kamaly-Asl is a full time paediatric neurosurgeon and Honorary Chair at Royal Manchester Children's Hospital. He trained in North Western Deanery with fellowships at Boston Children's Hospital and Sick Kids in Toronto. Ian is a member of council of The Royal College of Surgeons of England and The SBNS where he is lead for mentoring and tackling oppressive behaviours.

Peter Whitfield
University Hospitals Plymouth NHS Trust

Professor Peter Whitfield is a Consultant Neurosurgeon at the South West Neurosurgical Centre, University Hospitals Plymouth NHS Trust. His clinical interests include vascular neurosurgery, neuro oncology and trauma. He has held many roles in postgraduate neurosurgical education and is President of the Society of British Neurological Surgeons. Peter has published widely, and is passionate about education, training and the promotion of clinical research.

About the Series

Elements in Emergency Neurosurgery is intended for trainees and practitioners in Neurosurgery and Emergency Medicine as well as allied specialties all over the world. Authored by international experts, this series provides core knowledge, common clinical pathways and recommendations on the management of acute conditions of the brain and spine.

Cambridge Elements

Emergency Neurosurgery

Elements in the Series

Cranial and Spinal Tuberculosis Infections including Acute Presentations
Veekshith Shetty and Pragnesh Bhatt

Spinal Discitis and Epidural Abscess
Damjan Veljanoski and Pragnesh Bhatt

Adult Patient with Intraventricular, Paraventricular and Pineal Region Lesions
Mohamed Dablouk and Mahmoud Kamel

Ruptured Supratentorial Cerebral Artery Aneurysm with Large Intracerebral Haematoma
Samuel Hall and Diederik Bulters

Neurosurgical Handovers and Standards for Emergency Care
Simon Lammy and Jennifer Brown

Spontaneous Intracranial Haemorrhage Caused by a Non-aneurysmal Brain Vascular Malformation
Sherif R. W. Kirollos and Ramez W. Kirollos

Emergency Scenarios in Functional Neurosurgery
James Manfield and Nicholas Park

Management of a Patient with a Venous Sinus Thrombosis with or without an Intracerebral Haematoma
Helen Sims and James Choulerton

Patient with Suspected Cauda Equina Syndrome
Gabriel Metcalf-Cuenca and Patrick F. X. Statham

Assessment of a Patient in Coma
Alexander Shah and Holly Roy

Patient with Acute Thoracic Myelopathy due to Degenerative Disease
James M. W. Robins and Deb Pal

Management of Moderate or Severe Traumatic Brain Injury
Saeed Kayhanian, Erta Beqiri, Ari Ercole and Adel Helmy

A full series listing is available at: www.cambridge.org/EEMN

For EU product safety concerns, contact us at Calle de José Abascal, 56–1°, 28003 Madrid, Spain or eugpsr@cambridge.org.

www.ingramcontent.com/pod-product-compliance
Lightning Source LLC
LaVergne TN
LVHW021946060526
838200LV00042B/1936